Outbreak in the Wild

The Silent Threat of the Rabid Fox

Evelyn C. Kohl

Copyright

About the Author

In the fields of public health and epidemiology, Evelyn C. Kohl is a well-known person. Over the course of her 20-year career, She has become a top expert on infectious diseases and global health policy. She has a Ph.D. in public health from the well-known Johns Hopkins University and has done a lot of work for the World Health Organisation (WHO) and the Centres for Disease Control and Prevention (CDC).

Kohl's journey started with a strong desire to learn about and fight infectious diseases. In her early work, she did important studies on how different pathogens spread, which earned her a lot of praise and admiration in the scientific community. Over the years, she became more interested in putting effective public health plans into action, especially in areas that don't have enough resources.

Evelyn C. Kohl is an author who writes from a place of deep experience and knowledge. Her approach is characterized by a unique blend of scientific rigor and a deep empathy for the human situation. Koh lexpertly tells the story of a global health crisis in her latest book, "Outbreak In the wild," drawing on her vast knowledge and personal experiences.

She has made contributions beyond study and writing. She is also a respected teacher and mentor. She has been a professor at a number of top universities, where she has taught the next generation of public health workers. Her lectures and seminars are famous for their clarity, depth, and ability to inspire.

In "Outbreak In the wild, Evelyn not only provides an authoritative account of the pandemic but also dives into the societal and psychological effects of such global events. Her book is a testament to her commitment to improving public health and her belief in the power of educated action to create a better world.

Outside of her work endeavors, Evelyn is an avid traveler and a proponent of cultural exchange as a means to enhance global health understanding. Her experiences across different countries have enriched her perspective, which is evident in the global outlook of her work.

Evelyn C. Kohl's addition to the field of public health and her work in educating the public about the complexities of pandemics make her an invaluable voice in times of global health crises. Her book is not just a reflection of her vast knowledge but also a beacon of advice for a world navigating the uncertainties of future health challenges.

Table of Content

The Beginning....................................8

Chapter 1: The Rabies Virus................... 12

Chapter 2: Fox Behavior and Rabies.....22

Chapter 3: Transmission and Spread.....32

Chapter 4: Human and Animal
Interactions....................................42

Chapter 5: Rabies Prevention and
Control.. 52

Chapter 6: Case Studies......................... 62

Chapter 7: The Future of Rabies
Control.. 72

Conclusion.. 78

The Beginning

The Strange Case of the Wild Fox

The mysterious story of the mad fox can be found in the peaceful but wild parts of our world, where nature whispers wild secrets. People are both scared of and interested in this creature, which is often linked to folklore and stories from rural areas. With its strange appearance and unpredictable behaviour, the rabid fox is more than just a threat from old wives' tales. It is also a science mystery and a public health issue. In "Outbreak in the Wild: The Silent Threat of the Rabid Fox," we explore the strange world of these animals, trying to figure out what's really going on with them when they're rabid and what the bigger effects are on both the wild and the human world.

This trip isn't just about how a virus can make people sick; it's also a study of the complicated relationships between people and animals. It makes us think about the delicate balance that exists in our shared environments and makes us question where the lines are between the wild and the civilised. As we continue our journey, we learn not only about the fears and dangers of rabid foxes, but also about how strong nature is and how responsible we are as guardians of our planet.

Understanding Rabies: A Brief Overview

Rabies is a very old disease that has been known to people for thousands of years. The word "rabies" makes people think of crazy people and scary things. It is caused by a virus that attacks the central nervous system, leading to a series of neurological symptoms that almost usually result in death once they appear. This introduction provides a brief yet thorough overview of rabies, detailing its history, transmission, symptoms, and effect on both animal and human populations.

This section sets the stage for a deeper understanding of the disease, setting a foundation for the chapters that follow. It discusses the virus's mode of transmission, mainly through the saliva of infected animals, and its progression in the body, leading to the dramatic and often terrifying symptoms associated with the word "rabid." The overview also touches upon the global incidence of rabies, its effect on public health, and the efforts taken worldwide to control and prevent this deadly disease.

Chapter 1: The Rabies Virus

Origin and Nature of the Virus

Rabies, one of the oldest known zoonotic diseases, has haunted mankind and the animal kingdom for ages. This chapter dives into the origin and fundamental nature of the rabies virus, a pathogen surrounded by both historical dread and modern scientific inquiry.

The Ancient Scourge: Historical Perspective

The history of rabies is as old as civilization itself, with records of rabid animals going back to ancient Mesopotamia and Greece. This section explores how early societies viewed rabies, intertwining the virus's history with human culture, mythology, and medical understanding. It reflects on how rabies was often linked with supernatural forces due to its mysterious and frightening symptoms.

Virology of Rabies: Understanding the Pathogen

At the heart of this disease is the rabies virus, a part of the Lyssavirus genus. This section offers an in-depth look at the structure and life cycle of the rabies virus. It shows how the virus is uniquely adapted to invade the nervous system of mammals, leading to the severe neurological symptoms that mark the disease. The discussion includes the virus's method of transmission, mainly through saliva via bites, and its journey from the site of the bite to the brain.

Variants and Hosts: The Diversity of Rabies

Rabies is not a one-size-fits-all virus. This part of the chapter covers the different strains of the rabies virus, each adapted to specific animal hosts. The focus here is on the diversity of the virus and its ability to infect a wide range of animals, from domestic dogs to wild bats and, of course, foxes. This part also addresses the geographical distribution of different rabies strains, highlighting how the virus varies from one area to another.

Molecular Mechanism: How Rabies Hijacks the Body

Understanding the rabies virus also needs a look at its molecular mechanism – how it hijacks the host's nervous system. This section describes the process by which the virus enters nerve cells, replicates, and travels to the brain, causing encephalitis (inflammation of the brain). The discussion includes the biological reasons behind the notorious signs of rabies, such as hydrophobia (fear of water), aggression, and paralysis.

The Unseen Battle: The Host's Response

Despite being a potent pathogen, rabies often evades the immune system's initial defenses, allowing it to continue unnoticed until symptoms show. This part explains why rabies is so difficult to detect and treat once it has established itself in the host and why prevention through vaccination is important.

How Rabies Affects Mammals

The focus changes to understanding how the rabies virus affects mammals, giving a comprehensive view of the disease's progression, symptoms, and final impact on various species, including humans.

The Initial Invasion: Entry and Early Stages

Rabies starts its insidious journey in a mammal's body at the site of a bite from an infected animal. This part delves into the early stages of infection, where the virus enters muscle cells near the bite and starts its gradual move towards the peripheral nervous system. It outlines the initial viral replication process and the lack of major symptoms during this phase, which can last for weeks or even months.

Neurological Hijacking: The Journey to the Brain

One of the most important aspects of rabies infection is its progression through the nervous system to the brain. This part of the chapter explains how the virus travels along nerve cells, evading the immune system due to its protected pathway. The discussion highlights the mechanisms the virus uses to move within nerve cells and the reasons this journey can vary in length, affecting the incubation period of the disease.

Symptoms and Behavioral Changes

As the virus reaches the brain and starts to replicate rapidly, it causes severe inflammation and disruption of normal brain function. This part covers the array of symptoms that manifest in mammals, including standard signs like aggression, disorientation, excessive salivation, and hydrophobia. Behavioral changes in wild animals, such as loss of fear of people in foxes, are studied to understand how rabies can alter natural behaviors, leading to increased risk of transmission.

Species-Specific Responses

Different mammalian species show variations in their response to rabies infection. This part compares the disease's progression and impact in different animals, including domestic pets like dogs and cats, wildlife like foxes and bats, and humans. It discusses how the variability in symptoms and aggressiveness of the disease can depend on the species, and even on the individual strain of the rabies virus.

The Inevitable Outcome: Terminal Stage and Death

In the absence of intervention, rabies is almost invariably fatal once clinical symptoms show. This part offers a sobering look at the terminal stages of rabies, describing the rapid deterioration of neurological function leading to paralysis, coma, and death. It shows the reasons behind the high fatality rate and the importance of early post-exposure treatment in humans.

Impact on Ecosystems and Human Society

This discusses the ecological effect of rabies outbreaks in wildlife and the challenges they pose for conservation efforts. Additionally, the section discusses the significant public health concerns associated with rabies, especially in regions where vaccination and medical treatment are less available.

Through this detailed study of how rabies affects mammals, it provides a crucial basis for understanding the complexities and challenges of managing and preventing this deadly disease in both wild and domestic animals, as well as in human communities.

Chapter 2: Fox Behavior and Rabies

Normal vs. Rabid Fox Behavior

The attention shifts to the specific case of foxes, a key species in the study of rabies. This chapter aims to contrast the typical behaviors of healthy foxes against those exhibited by foxes infected with rabies, giving insights into how the disease alters their natural behavior.

Understanding Normal Fox Behavior

To recognise the changes wrought by rabies, it is necessary first to understand the typical behaviors and characteristics of healthy foxes. This part introduces the reader to the natural habits of foxes, including their social structures, hunting practices, and territory marking behaviors. It shows how foxes, known for their cunning and adaptability, interact with their environment and other species, including humans. The discussion also hits on the variations in behavior among different species of foxes, such as red foxes, gray foxes, and arctic foxes.

The Onset of Rabies: Early Behavioral Changes

When a fox contracts rabies, the initial stages of the infection may not quickly alter its behavior. This section describes the subtle changes that might occur as the virus starts to affect the fox's nervous system. It discusses the challenges in detecting rabies in its early stages, especially in wild populations where close observation is not feasible.

Dramatic Behavioral Shifts: Signs of Rabid Foxes

As the rabies virus progresses to the brain, it causes major changes in a fox's behavior. This part of the chapter details the more noticeable and often alarming signs of rabid foxes. These include increased aggression, loss of fear of humans, disorientation, erratic movements, and the typical excessive drooling or foaming at the mouth due to trouble swallowing. The section emphasizes how these behavioral changes increase the likelihood of the rabid fox coming into contact with people and other animals, thereby facilitating the spread of the virus.

Danger to Humans and Other Animals

This section discusses the direct threat that rabid foxes pose to humans, pets, and livestock. It discusses the risk of rabies transmission through bites or scratches and the importance of public knowledge in areas where rabid foxes are present. The discussion includes guidelines on what to do when encountering a possibly rabid fox and the necessary steps to take in the event of exposure.

Conservation and Management Challenges

This concludes by examining the effect of rabies on fox populations and the wider ecosystem. It discusses the challenges faced in managing rabid fox outbreaks, especially in balancing disease control with conservation efforts. This part also explores the strategies used by wildlife officials to monitor and control rabies in fox populations, such as vaccination programs and public education campaigns.

By contrasting normal fox behavior with the altered states induced by rabies, This provides a complete understanding of the profound effects of this disease on individual animals and the cascading impacts on wildlife and human communities.

Recognizing the Signs of Rabies in Foxes

This section is crucial for knowing how to identify rabies in foxes, which is pivotal for both public safety and effective wildlife management. Recognizing the signs of rabies in these animals is challenging yet important, as it helps in early intervention and preventing the spread of the disease.

1 Physical Symptoms of Rabies in Foxes

By detailing the physical symptoms that may suggest a fox is suffering from rabies. These signs include:

- Excessive drooling or foaming at the mouth, indicative of trouble swallowing.

- Weakness or partial weakness, particularly of the hind legs.

- Unkempt appearance due to neglect of normal grooming practices.

- Visible confusion or staggering, suggesting neurological impairment.

2 Behavioral Indicators of Rabid Foxes

The behavioral changes in rabid foxes are often more marked than the physical symptoms. This part of the chapter focuses on these changes, which include:

- Loss of fear of people, leading to abnormally bold behavior.

- Uncharacteristic aggression, such as attacking items, other animals, or people without provocation.

- Nocturnal animals like foxes being busy during the day.

- Unusual vocalizations or a total lack of fear in situations that would normally cause distress.

3 The Progression of Symptoms

Understanding the progression of rabies symptoms in foxes is important for identifying and reacting to potential cases.

Importance of Caution and Professional Assessment

This emphasizes the importance of exercising caution around foxes showing potential signs of rabies. It advises against approaching or trying to capture a suspected rabid fox, instead recommending calling local wildlife authorities or animal control professionals. The role of these professionals in safely assessing and handling possibly rabid animals.

1   Differential Diagnosis: Separating Rabies from Other Conditions

Rabies is not the only condition that can cause behavioral or physical changes in foxes. This part covers other illnesses and conditions that may mimic rabies symptoms, underlining the importance of professional diagnosis. It also touches on the methods used by wildlife experts and vets to confirm a rabies infection, such as observation of symptoms and laboratory testing.

2 Public Awareness and Reporting

The importance of general awareness in recognizing and reporting potential rabies cases. It stresses the role of community vigilance in rabies surveillance and control, and how educating the public about the signs of rabies in wildlife adds to overall ecosystem health and public safety.

Chapter 3: Transmission and Spread

How Rabies Spreads Among Wildlife

The focus turns to the dynamics of rabies transmission among wildlife populations, especially how the virus spreads and the factors that influence its movement through different animal communities.

Understanding the Transmission Cycle

The chapter starts by explaining the basic transmission cycle of rabies among wildlife. It details how the rabies virus is mainly spread through saliva, usually via bites from infected animals. This section provides a clear explanation of how the virus can pass from one animal to another, stressing that the exchange of saliva through biting is the most common mode of transmission.

Species as Carriers and Vectors

Different species play varying parts in the spread of rabies. This part of the chapter discusses the idea of "reservoir species" — animals that are primary carriers of the virus and are responsible for maintaining the virus within an ecosystem. It studies how species like bats, raccoons, skunks, and foxes act as reservoirs for the rabies virus and how their behaviors and interactions facilitate the spread of the disease within and across species.

Behavioral Factors in Transmission

Behavior plays a significant part in the transmission of rabies. This section delves into how the altered behavior of rabid animals, such as increased aggression and loss of fear, adds to the spread of the virus. It also discusses the role of territorial and mating behaviors in the transmission dynamics, especially in species like foxes, where fights and mating can result in bites and virus spread.

Geographical and Environmental Influences

The geographical spread of rabies is influenced by different environmental factors. This part of the chapter studies how landscape features, human activity, and ecological changes can affect the movement of rabies through wildlife populations. It also studies how human encroachment into wildlife habitats can increase the interactions between rabid animals and people or domestic animals.

The Role of Migratory and Transient Species

Migratory and transient species can act as vectors for rabies, spreading the virus across long distances. This section looks at the role of these species in spreading rabies to new areas and discusses how human activities like the relocation of animals can unknowingly contribute to the wider dissemination of the virus.

Impact of Climate Change and Ecosystem Dynamics

The final part of the chapter discusses the broader implications of climate change and ecosystem dynamics on the transmission of rabies. It explains how changes in climate and habitat can alter the behaviors and ranges of wildlife, possibly leading to increased rabies transmission. This section underscores the importance of knowing and adapting to these changes in the context of rabies management and control.

The Role of Foxes in the Rabies Ecosystem

This discussion zeroes in on the specific role that foxes play in the rabies ecosystem, stressing their importance in the transmission and dynamics of the disease.

1 Foxes as a Reservoir Species

This starts by establishing foxes as a key reservoir species for the rabies virus in many ecosystems. It explains what it means to be a reservoir species, emphasizing how fox populations can harbor and support the virus over extended periods, sometimes even when the disease is not actively manifesting in epidemic proportions.

2 Transmission Dynamics in Fox Populations

Here, this dives into the specific ways rabies is transmitted within fox populations. This includes detailing behaviors unique to foxes that enable the spread of rabies, such as their social hierarchy, territorial disputes, and mating behaviors. The discussion also covers the density of fox populations and how it affects the spread rate of rabies.

3 Foxes and the Cross-Species Transmission

Foxes often interact with other wildlife species as well as domestic animals, making them important players in the cross-species transmission of rabies. This section explores these interactions and the role of foxes in spreading rabies to other species, including domestic dogs, cats, and livestock. It also touches on the effects of these transmissions on public health and the wider ecosystem.

4   Geographical   Variability   in Fox-Related Rabies

The incidence and characteristics of rabies can vary greatly in fox populations based on geographic location. This part of the chapter explores these variations, discussing how factors like species of foxes (e.g., red foxes vs. gray foxes), local climate, and habitat types affect the prevalence and nature of rabies in different areas.

Control and Management Strategies in Fox Populations

Controlling rabies in fox populations offers unique challenges and opportunities. This section describes the strategies employed to manage and reduce rabies in these animals, including oral rabies vaccination programs, public education, and wildlife monitoring efforts. It shows successful case studies and the ongoing challenges faced in different parts of the world.

Foxes as Sentinels in Rabies Surveillance

The role of foxes as sentinel species in rabies tracking. It shows how monitoring rabies in fox populations can provide early warning signs of outbreaks and help in assessing the effectiveness of rabies control methods in broader wildlife and domestic animal populations.

By focusing on the role of foxes in the rabies ecosystem, this part of the chapter offers a detailed look at the complexities involved in understanding and managing this disease in a key wildlife species, underscoring their significance in the overall dynamics of rabies in nature.

Chapter 4: Human and Animal Interactions

Cases of Rabid Foxes and Human Encounters

This shifts to the interface between people, animals, and the rabies virus, focusing especially on the interactions between humans and rabid foxes. This chapter aims to put light on the realities, risks, and outcomes of such encounters.

Documenting Human-Fox Encounters

By presenting different documented cases of human encounters with rabid foxes. These narratives offer real-world insights into how such interactions occur, the risks involved, and the effects for both the humans and the foxes. This section may include accounts from rural and urban settings, highlighting the diverse contexts in which people may come into contact with rabid wildlife.

Analysis of Encounter Scenarios

This part looks deeper into the dynamics of human-fox encounters. It analyzes common scenarios, such as foxes entering residential areas, attacks on people, and incidents involving pets. The discussion aims to understand the factors that lead to these encounters, such as habitat encroachment, changes in fox behavior due to rabies, and human activities that accidentally attract or provoke foxes.

Public Health Implications

Here, the focus is on the public health consequences of encounters with rabid foxes. It addresses the risk of rabies transmission to people, the necessary medical response to potential rabies exposure, and the psychological effect of such encounters. This section also discusses the broader public health challenges faced by rabies in wildlife, especially in regions where the disease is endemic.

Preventive Measures and Best Practices

Preventing encounters with rabid foxes and managing them safely when they do occur is important. This section offers guidelines and best practices for avoiding encounters with potentially rabid wildlife, what to do if an encounter happens, and how to safely and humanely deal with rabid or suspected rabid foxes. It includes advice for homeowners, outdoor enthusiasts, and professionals who may encounter these animals in the course of their job.

Community Education and Awareness

The chapter emphasizes the importance of community education and awareness in avoiding and safely managing encounters with rabid foxes. It highlights successful public education campaigns and strategies for raising knowledge about rabies risks, wildlife behavior, and responsible coexistence with wildlife.

Role of Local Authorities and Wildlife Agencies

The part discusses the role of local authorities, public health officials, and wildlife agencies in managing the interface between humans, animals, and rabies. This includes their duties in responding to incidents of rabid fox encounters, controlling rabies in wildlife populations, and educating the public.

Safety Measures and Preventing Rabies Transmission

Outlining comprehensive safety measures and strategies to prevent the transmission of rabies, particularly in the context of potential human and fox interactions.

1 **Understanding the Risk**

Before delving into specific measures, the section starts with an explanation of the risks associated with rabies transmission from foxes to humans. This includes understanding how rabies is transmitted, finding situations that might increase the risk of exposure, and recognizing the importance of preventive actions.

2 **Vaccination: The First Line of Defense**

Vaccination is highlighted as the most effective preventive step against rabies. The talk covers the importance of vaccinating pets, such as dogs and cats, and the role of wildlife vaccination programs, particularly oral rabies vaccination efforts targeting fox populations.

3 Educating the Public on Safe Behavior

Education is a key component in avoiding rabies transmission. This part focuses on educating the public about safe behaviors around wildlife, including keeping a safe distance from wild animals, supervising pets outdoors, and securing food sources that might attract foxes or other wildlife to residential areas.

4 Immediate Actions Following Potential Exposure

The section offers detailed guidance on what to do in the event of a potential rabies exposure, such as a bite or scratch from a fox. It stresses the importance of immediate wound care, seeking medical attention, and the necessity of post-exposure prophylaxis (PEP) for rabies.

5 Managing Wildlife Encounters

Advice on managing encounters with wildlife, especially foxes, is given here. It includes tips on deterring foxes from entering residential areas, humanely dealing with fox sightings, and the importance of not trying to capture or handle wild animals.

6 Collaboration with Health and Wildlife Authorities

The value of collaboration between public health authorities, wildlife agencies, and the community is explored. This part explains how these entities work together in monitoring rabies cases, responding to wildlife encounters, and implementing rabies control measures.

7 Legal and Ethical Considerations

This part discusses the legal and ethical considerations in dealing with rabid or suspected rabid animals. It covers the laws and regulations governing wildlife management and the ethical considerations in humane wildlife treatment.

8 Preparedness and Response Plans

Lastly, the chapter talks about the value of having preparedness and response plans for potential rabies outbreaks. This includes community-level plans involving public health departments, wildlife agencies, and other stakeholders to successfully react to and manage rabies incidents.

By addressing these various aspects of safety measures and rabies transmission prevention, this part of Chapter 4 provides essential information and guidelines for minimizing the risk of rabies transmission and ensuring safe interactions between humans and wildlife.

Chapter 5: Rabies Prevention and Control

Vaccination Programs for Wildlife and Domestic Animals

The focus moves to proactive measures in rabies prevention and control, with a significant emphasis on vaccination programs for both wildlife and domestic animals. This chapter aims to highlight the importance, challenges, and successes of these vaccination attempts.

The Role of Vaccination in Rabies Control

The chapter starts by establishing the fundamental role that vaccination plays in controlling and preventing rabies. It explains how vaccinations work to provide immunity against the virus and outlines the reasoning behind targeting both domestic animals and wildlife in comprehensive rabies control strategies.

Vaccination Programs for Domestic Animals

This part delves into the vaccination programs for domestic animals, mainly dogs and cats, which are often the bridge between wildlife rabies and humans. The talk covers the importance of regular vaccination schedules, the impact these programs have had on public health, and the difficulties in ensuring widespread coverage, especially in rural or underserved areas.

Oral Rabies Vaccination (ORV) for Wildlife

One of the most important advances in wildlife rabies control is the development of oral rabies vaccines. This part of the chapter focuses on ORV programs, especially those targeting fox populations. It discusses the methodology of distributing edible vaccine baits, the success of these programs in reducing rabies cases in wildlife, and the logistical challenges involved in implementing ORV campaigns.

Case Studies: Successes and Lessons Learned

This section shows various case studies from around the world where vaccination programs have successfully controlled or eliminated rabies. Examples may include the elimination of rabies in fox populations in certain European countries or successful ORV projects in North America. The lessons learned from these case studies provide valuable insights for future rabies control attempts.

Innovations in Vaccine Development and Distribution

The chapter also explores ongoing study and innovations in the field of rabies vaccine development and distribution methods. This includes advancements in vaccine efficacy, the creation of new delivery methods for wildlife, and the use of technology and data in planning and monitoring vaccination campaigns.

Collaboration and Multisectoral Approaches

The value of collaboration across different sectors is emphasized in this part of the chapter. It highlights how government agencies, public health officials, wildlife groups, and communities nccd to work together for effective rabies control. The role of international organizations and cross-border cooperation in managing rabies in transboundary wildlife populations is also explored.

Challenges and Future Directions

The chapter concludes with a discussion on the ongoing challenges in rabies prevention and control, such as funding limitations, accessibility problems in remote areas, and general awareness and compliance. It also looks ahead to the future directions of rabies control efforts, considering new challenges like climate change and habitat alteration.

Public Health Measures and Awareness

Public health measures and awareness campaigns play in the prevention and control of rabies. It highlights the strategies and efforts aimed at reducing the risk of rabies in human populations.

1 Surveillance and Monitoring

By discussing the importance of surveillance and monitoring systems in public health. It explains how tracking rabies cases in both animals and people helps authorities to identify outbreak areas, monitor trends, and allocate resources effectively. This part includes examples of successful surveillance systems and the use of technology in tracking rabies.

2 Educational Campaigns and Community Outreach

One of the most successful tools in rabies prevention is public education. This covers the different educational campaigns and community outreach programs designed to increase awareness about rabies. It discusses how these programs teach the public about rabies transmission, symptoms, and preventive measures, including responsible pet ownership and avoiding contact with wild animals.

3 Collaboration with Veterinary Services

The collaboration between public health and veterinary services is important for effective rabies control. This section shows how these two sectors work together to ensure widespread vaccination of domestic animals, educate pet owners, and manage stray animal populations.

4 Post-Exposure Prophylaxis (PEP) and Medical Resources

Access to post-exposure prophylaxis (PEP) is a key aspect of rabies prevention in humans. This part discusses the procedures for administering PEP, the challenges of ensuring availability and affordability of rabies vaccines and immunoglobulins for humans, and the efforts to improve access to these lifesaving treatments.

5 Policy and Legislation

Effective rabies control also includes supportive policy and legislation. This part studies the laws and regulations related to rabies control, such as mandatory pet vaccination, regulations for importing animals, and guidelines for managing rabies outbreaks.

6 Community Participation and Empowerment

The importance of community involvement in rabies prevention attempts is underscored in this part of the chapter. It discusses how empowering communities to take active roles, from reporting stray or sick animals to participating in vaccination drives, enhances the success of rabies control programs.

7   Addressing Cultural Beliefs and Practices

This section acknowledges the effect of cultural beliefs and practices on rabies control efforts. It explores how educational efforts can respectfully address and integrate cultural perspectives to improve community engagement and compliance with rabies prevention measures.

By comprehensively addressing public health measures and awareness, this underscores the multi-faceted approach needed to effectively manage and reduce the threat of rabies in human populations.

Chapter 6: Case Studies

Documented Incidents Involving Rabid Foxes

Series of case studies that look into specific, documented incidents involving rabid foxes. These case studies provide real-world examples that show the diverse aspects of rabies transmission, public health implications, and the effectiveness of control methods.

1 Incident Analysis and Context

Each case study starts with a detailed analysis of a specific incident involving a rabid fox. The context of the incident, including geographical location, time of year, and the environmental setting, is given to give readers a comprehensive understanding of the situation.

2 Human-Fox Interactions

This part of the case studies focuses on incidents where rabid foxes have interacted with humans. It covers the circumstances of these encounters, the immediate actions taken by the people involved, and the following public health response. These narratives try to highlight the risks of rabies transmission to humans and the importance of awareness and preventive steps.

3 Fox-to-Domestic Animal Transmission

Some case studies examine situations where rabid foxes have come into touch with domestic animals, such as pets or livestock.

4 Outbreak Scenarios

Several case studies focus on outbreaks of rabies within fox populations, showing how the disease can spread rapidly in certain conditions. These examples describe the response by wildlife and public health authorities, the challenges faced, and the outcomes of intervention efforts.

Success Stories in Rabies Control

To provide a balanced view, this also includes case studies that show successful rabies control and prevention efforts. These might include successful vaccination campaigns, effective public education projects, or instances where potential outbreaks were successfully contained.

Lessons Learned

Each case study ends with a section on the lessons learned from the incident. This includes insights into better disease surveillance, public health strategies, wildlife management practices, and community education approaches.

Global Perspectives

Recognizing the global nature of rabies, the case studies include events from different parts of the world. This approach provides a wider understanding of how rabies impacts diverse ecosystems and cultures and the various strategies employed globally to fight the disease.

By presenting these case studies, It offers useful insights into the real-world challenges and successes in managing rabies in fox populations and the effects for wildlife, domestic animals, and human health. These narratives serve to teach, inform, and guide future efforts in rabies prevention and control.

Analysis and Lessons Learned

Comprehensive analysis of the documented incidents involving rabid foxes, drawing out key lessons learned from these case studies. This analysis aims to synthesize the insights gained and to guide future strategies for rabies control and prevention.

Identifying Patterns and Common Challenges

This part of the chapter examines any recurring patterns or common challenges noticed across the different case studies. It looks at aspects like common transmission vectors, typical environmental conditions conducive to outbreaks, and frequent problems in public health reactions. This analysis helps in understanding the critical factors that lead to rabies incidents involving foxes.

Effectiveness of Response Strategies

Here, the chapter assesses the effectiveness of different response strategies applied in the documented cases. This includes evaluating the influence of vaccination programs, the efficiency of public health responses to human and animal exposures, and the effectiveness of community awareness efforts. The aim is to identify what worked well and what could be improved in future replies.

Public Health and Safety Implications

This part draws out the broader public health and safety implications from the case studies. It discusses how these incidents have affected communities, the psychological impact on people involved, and the economic consequences of rabies outbreaks. The section also reflects on the value of proactive public health steps in preventing such incidents.

Advancements in Rabies Research and Management

Based on the case studies, this part highlights any advancements in rabies research and management techniques. It explores new findings in rabies transmission, vaccine development, and wildlife management methods that have emerged from these real-world scenarios.

1 Community Involvement and Education

One of the key lessons often drawn from rabies cases is the crucial role of community involvement and education. This section emphasizes the need for ongoing public education about rabies risks and prevention, as well as community involvement in rabies surveillance and control efforts.

2 Policy and Legislation Recommendations

Drawing from the lessons learned, this part offers suggestions for policy and legislative changes to better manage and prevent rabies outbreaks. This may include ideas for improving wildlife management policies, enhancing rabies surveillance systems, or updating public health guidelines.

3 Preparing for Future Challenges

Finally, the chapter ends with insights into preparing for future challenges in rabies control, especially considering factors like climate change, urbanization, and changes in wildlife populations. It shows the importance of adaptive management and resilience in public health planning to address the evolving nature of rabies risks.

By providing a thorough analysis and extracting lessons learned from various case studies, this section adds significantly to the body of knowledge on rabies management and prevention, offering valuable guidance for future efforts to fight this enduring public health threat.

Chapter 7: The Future of Rabies Control

Strategies for Wildlife and Ecosystem Health

This part of the chapter outlines approaches and practices that not only target rabies but also add to the overall well-being of wildlife populations and their habitats.

1 Balancing Rabies Control with Conservation

The chapter starts by discussing the need to balance rabies control efforts with wildlife conservation. It emphasizes tactics that reduce rabies transmission in wildlife without negatively impacting species populations or biodiversity. This includes considerations of ethical and humane treatment of animals in rabies control efforts.

2 Habitat Management and Preservation

Effective habitat management plays a critical role in keeping healthy wildlife populations and reducing rabies risks. This part explores how preserving natural habitats and maintaining ecological balance can avoid the conditions that lead to increased rabies transmission, such as overpopulation or unhealthy animal densities.

3   Ecosystem-Based   Management Approaches

This part of the chapter delves into ecosystem-based management methods that consider the interactions between different species and their environments. It explains how these approaches can help in monitoring and controlling rabies spread, while also supporting overall ecosystem health.

4 Integrating Public Health and Wildlife Management

The integration of public health and wildlife management is important for effective rabies control. This section outlines how joint efforts between these areas can lead to more comprehensive and effective strategies. It shows the importance of interdisciplinary collaboration and shared knowledge in managing health risks at the human-wildlife interface.

5   Community Engagement and Education

Engaging local communities in wildlife and ecosystem health is important. This section discusses the importance of community education programs that foster coexistence with wildlife, promote understanding of rabies risks, and encourage involvement in rabies prevention and wildlife conservation efforts.

Innovative Technologies in Wildlife Monitoring

Advancements in technology offer new possibilities for wildlife monitoring and rabies surveillance. The chapter examines how tools like GPS tracking, drones, and remote sensing can provide valuable data on wildlife movements and health, adding to more effective rabies control and ecosystem management.

Adapting to Climate Change and Environmental Shifts

This addresses the need to adapt rabies control strategies in reaction to climate change and environmental shifts. It explores how changing climates and habitats can change wildlife behavior and rabies transmission patterns, underscoring the need for flexible and adaptive management strategies.

By focusing on strategies for wildlife and ecosystem health, this highlights the interconnectedness of rabies control with broader environmental and conservation problems. It underscores the importance of a holistic approach that protects both public health and the health of our planet's ecosystems.

Conclusion

The Continuing Challenge of Rabies

The concluding chapter of "Outbreak in the Wild: The Silent Threat of the Rabid Fox" focuses on the enduring challenge that rabies presents to public health, wildlife management, and global communities. This section reiterates the complex nature of rabies as a disease that not only affects individual health but also has larger implications for ecological and societal well-being. It emphasizes the ongoing necessity for vigilance, study, and innovative approaches to control and finally eradicate this ancient scourge.

Persistent Threats and Evolving Challenges

Despite significant advances in understanding and managing rabies, the virus continues to pose a serious threat, especially in areas with limited access to vaccines and healthcare. It addresses the evolving challenges in rabies control, such as urbanization, climate change, and changes in wildlife populations and habitats.

Global Impact and the Need for Unified Efforts

The global effect of rabies is underscored, stressing the need for a unified, international effort in addressing this disease. The conclusion calls for continued collaboration between countries, organizations, and disciplines to share knowledge, resources, and strategies to combat rabies successfully.

The Role of Education and Awareness in Rabies Prevention

1   Education as a Cornerstone of Prevention

This part of the conclusion emphasizes the important role of education in rabies prevention. It underscores the importance of raising knowledge about rabies transmission, symptoms, and prevention methods, especially in communities at higher risk of rabies exposure.

2   Empowering Communities Through Knowledge

The power of education to empower communities is discussed, highlighting how educated individuals and groups are better equipped to take preventive measures, seek timely medical care, and support rabies control initiatives. The section stresses the need for ongoing educational campaigns that are culturally sensitive and available to diverse populations.

3   Role of Media and Technology in Awareness

It discusses how innovative use of digital platforms, social media, and traditional media can successfully disseminate information and engage broader audiences in rabies education and prevention efforts.

In ending, the book makes a call for continued action against rabies. It encourages readers to remain informed and involved, and to support efforts in rabies research, public health initiatives, and wildlife conservation. The conclusion reaffirms the view that with collective and sustained efforts, the goal of a rabies-free future is achievable.

www.ingramcontent.com/pod-product-compliance
Lightning Source LLC
Chambersburg PA
CBHW050839260726

48660CB00006B/2334